THE
MEETING

For the Families & Friends of Alcoholics

Book 2

THE
MEETING

For the Families & Friends of Alcoholics

Book 2

Lois Barleycorn Dickens

authorHOUSE®

AuthorHouse™
1663 Liberty Drive
Bloomington, IN 47403
www.authorhouse.com
Phone: 1-800-839-8640

Published by AuthorHouse   06/06/2012

ISBN: 978-1-4685-8261-1 (sc)
ISBN: 978-1-4685-8262-8 (e)

For the Loved Ones of Alcoholics

To A & H—they know who they are.

The Meetings

Meeting 4   Courage 1

Meeting 5   One Day at a Time 24

Meeting 6   Looking for Help? 48

Meeting 4

Tonight's Topic—Courage

AL stands for Alcoholics' Loved Ones and is a meeting for anyone who is, or has been, affected by someone else's drinking, regardless of whether the person is still drinking or not.

ALICE says,

"Shall we make a start everybody?

One of the disciplines in AL is we start on time and we finish on time, regardless.

So, I will read the suggested opening:

We would like to welcome you to this AL meeting.

The AL meeting is a group of relatives and friends of problem drinkers who share their experience, strength and hope in order to solve their common problems. We believe alcoholism is a family illness and that changed attitudes can aid recovery.

I would like to welcome you all to this AL meeting and although we have no newcomers here tonight I would still like us to go round the room and introduce ourselves, using first names only because it takes us all a little time to remember everybody's name."

Meet the Group

ALICE

"Hello, my name is Alice and I am chairing the meeting tonight. It is our son who has a problem with alcohol. My husband Jeff is here with me tonight."

EDDIE

"I'm Eddie and as most of you know I'm an alcoholic. I'm a recovering alcoholic myself and I'm also married to a recovering alcoholic so I qualify for membership of AL as I have a family member who is alcohol dependent. I am the main sharer for tonight."

STAVROS

"I'm Stavros. My ex-wife was the drinker and trying to live with the impact that had on my own life brought me into this group."

CLARISSA

"Hello, I'm Clarissa and the alcoholic in my life is my husband but I am here tonight for me."

VICKY

"Hello, I'm Vicky and the problem drinker in my life is my daughter."

JEFF

"My name is Jeff and the person with the drink problem in our life is our son. He is still drinking and is drunk most days."

KALEB

"Hello, I'm Kaleb and the alcoholic in my life is my wife, who is currently trying to give up alcohol without the help of any support group."

PIPPA

"Hello, I'm Pippa and I'm here tonight because I really need the on-going support I can get from the group."

MACK

"Hi, I'm Mack and it's my son who is addicted to alcohol."

ELSA

"Hello I'm Elsa and I am a long time member of the group and it is my father who is the alcoholic in my life".

* * *

ALICE

"Can I remind everyone that this is an anonymous group and we use first names only. Anonymity is one of the key principles we adhere to in the group. You do not need to tell us who you are, where you live, where you work, what you do—absolutely nothing about your personal details at all if you don't want to.

There are 10 of us here tonight but the numbers vary each week and sometimes there are more of us and sometimes less.

You don't have to come every week but we do suggest you attend as regularly as you can if you want to benefit from what's on offer here. Our only purpose is to share our experience, strength and hope to help ourselves and each other to gain some peace of mind because our lives have been affected by an alcohol dependent person. Anything else about your life is no concern of ours unless you choose to share it with us.

So, as I've said my name is Alice and although I am chairing the meeting tonight, next time someone else will be chairing because we practice the principle of rotation of leadership in the group.

A special word for our recent members, it may all still seem strange and you will probably go away not understanding much about what you hear tonight but if you feel something that brings you back then that is enough to be going on with. Just keep coming back and it will eventually start to become much clearer about what support you can gain from the group.

Also, although we meet up in a church hall this programme is not religious and has no connection to any church. The only reason we meet here is because of low costs.

So on with the meeting.

Every week we have a different theme and tonight's theme is:

Courage

Jeff can you start us off with the 12 steps please?"

JEFF

"**Step 1**: We admitted we were powerless over the problem drinker and that our lives had become unmanageable."

KALEB

"**Step 2**: We came to believe that a power greater than ourselves could restore us to serenity."

PIPPA

"**Step 3**: We made a decision to turn our will and our lives over to the care of our higher power (HP)."

MACK

"**Step 4**: We made a searching and fearless moral inventory of ourselves."

ELSA

"**Step 5**: We admitted to our HP, to ourselves and to another human being the exact nature of our wrongs."

ALICE

"**Step 6**: We were entirely ready to have our HP remove all these defects of character."

EDDIE

"**Step 7**: We humbly asked our HP to remove our shortcomings."

STAVROS

"**Step 8**: We made a list of all persons we had harmed and became willing to make amends to them all."

CLARISSA

"**Step 9**: We made direct amends to such people wherever possible, except when to do so would injure them or others."

VICKY

"**Step 10**: We continued to take personal inventory and when we were wrong promptly admitted it."

JEFF

"**Step 11**: We sought through reflection and meditation to improve our conscious contact with our HP, seeking only knowledge of our HP's will for us and the power to carry that out."

<u>KALEB</u>

"**Step 12**: Having had an emotional and spiritual awakening as the result of these Steps, we tried to carry this message to others, and to practice these principles in all our affairs."

*   *   *

<u>ALICE</u>

"Eddie has agreed to be our main sharer for tonight.

Also can I just remind you there is no obligation for anyone to chair or share.

You can remain silent and just listen if you prefer but those who do decide to share are allowed to do so without interruption from others.

So over to you Eddie, on the theme of— **Courage**."

Eddie is a recovering alcoholic and has been a member of AA for 20 years. He has been sober for 18 years. He is a semi-retired university lecturer. He joined AL over 18 months ago because he is married to Sarah, who is also a recovering alcoholic.

<u>EDDIE</u>

"Thank you everyone for being here tonight.

Well for me courage and fear sort of go together like two sides of the same coin really. I find if I face my fear, my courage grows as well.

When I came into this group I think I came with an advantage and a disadvantage. As an alcoholic myself I always wanted to run away from everything that was threatening but I also had the advantage of having worked a 12 step programme before in AA so it wasn't a complete surprise to me.

When I first stumbled into AA I was totally unhappy, miserable and a drunk. My life had become mainly about pleasure seeking all the time just to keep me afloat but it was just a type of survival existence—it wasn't a life. I had a belief that I just had to keep up an act and hope nobody could see through me and it was very hard work. So hard that I needed a drink to escape from the mental and physical exhaustion of it all. Looking back I suppose I was just like a very, very frightened child-like person.

In AA, I very soon realised it was all about me having to change and that was a very frightening thought. I didn't know what kind of change it would be but I knew it would have to be something pretty major to keep me off the booze. Anyway I went to AA and I started to listen to people and I realised it was a bit like setting off on a journey through the jungle with a machete and you have to hack a pathway through but fortunately there were a lot of other people who had travelled that way before and the pathway was already laid out for me if I wanted it. So I had two choices—I could follow those who had gone before or I could try to make my own way through the jungle. Fortunately, I wasn't so arrogant to think I could do it my way so I followed what others had done and low and behold it worked. I think the main problem had been my own thinking, it was the way it was and I had never thought to question it.

People said I would have to find out what was wrong with me and put it right. If I had gone into AA before I reached that rock bottom stage I would have been saying—'who the hell do they think they are to even suggest there is anything wrong with me!' But thankfully I had hit a brick wall so that stopped me in my tracks, so I had to find some other way than just trying to sort it out myself.

So when I came to AL, I also wanted to run away. My alcoholism never goes away, it's always lurking—some people call it our default setting, so anything that's threatening, I will want to run away from. However, because I have been through this change before with the 12 Steps in AA, I realised it was the same 12 Steps even though I wasn't quite sure how it was going to apply to me living with an alcoholic.

Nevertheless I just accepted it and it was a great advantage to me not to have totally new stuff to deal with which I didn't understand.

I just listened to what people said with an open-mind and I was helped because I could identify with what people were saying. I think we can't and we don't know what has brought us here because we do what we have always done and we thought that was right and we never questioned it.

In those early days in AA, I think my ego just wanted to manipulate the programme for my own ends and so I kept having 'slips', for the newcomers that's just an expression we use to say we have started drinking again. Anyway, I think I wanted to pick and choose which bits of the programme I could use mainly so people couldn't see through me. I didn't have any hang-up's about having a HP—I was already open to that because I had experienced glimpses of a type of spiritual awakening because something always seemed to draw me to where I needed to be. People often joked about me having a guardian angel because I had walked out of so many situations that really no one should have survived—but I did. So I had it at the back of my mind that some sort of power was watching out for me because I certainly wasn't watching out for myself when I was blacking out through drink.

Oh, and just for the record all you good people sitting here tonight who have tried or are still trying to stop the alcoholics in your life from drinking—just pack it in, because you'll never win that one. An alcoholic's self-will is made of cast-iron which has been built up over years of living in a perceived war-zone where everyone is the enemy, even you, so trying to break their Will is useless—they would rather die. In my own case—nobody would have got me to come into this programme until I was ready to come. I was stubborn in the extreme and such was my thinking that nobody could have got me to go to AA before I was ready to go.

The definition for stubbornness in the dictionary should read 'alcoholic thinking' because when someone tried to control my self-will the sparks would fly, the nastiness would come in and the battle would commence—it was warfare really. So that's what you are faced with if you have an alcoholic in your life. Even in the early days of sobriety and working a 12 Step Programme it takes a good while for an alcoholic to recover from these self-sabotaging attitudes they have. My faulty thinking made me believe I was always fighting for my life and I couldn't give in because the fear was too great.

All my life I had felt fear, totally all-consuming fear. I never felt safe. I always felt as if I was on my own, so this looming sense of shouldering all that responsibility for everything was too much to bear. I was always wary, always thinking, 'Oh I'm on my own in the world nobody is going to look out for me'. It was an awful and crazy way to live.

Happily all of that changed when I first walked into AA and I can still remember those people who were there for me all those years ago, they were fantastic! I had finally found a place I could go where I could get help. I could off-load things which I had been bottling up for years.

The sort of person I was then was a person full of secrets and I was basically living a lie because I thought I couldn't afford to be truthful with my wife or anybody else in my life. I was behaving badly in my personal life. In my working life, I thought one of these days they would catch me out because I never felt good enough to be doing the job I was doing. Yet nobody ever complained about my work, it was just the way I thought and felt about myself—it was all in my own head.

I think as time went on in the programme I realised the whole business of working the Steps and emptying out that enormous rubbish bin full of stuff I had held inside for years was very important for me. When I said I was living a lie—I meant I had all of these secrets and they were festering away inside of me affecting how I behaved towards everybody else in my life. The way I behaved towards my wife, my children, my family, work friends, everyone and everything was awful because my fear never went away and it stopped me doing what other people do.

9

Today I don't have those secrets and life is so much easier for me. I feel as though I can participate in life, which in the drinking days and the first few years afterwards I couldn't. When I wasn't participating I was just sort of waiting for something to happen and I didn't know what. I think it was the constant fear that my wife would leave me – and in the end she did.

So as time goes on it's about living an open life, participating more in life. I've made amends to my sister who I didn't speak to for over 10 years—so that's a major achievement for me. I haven't been able to make amends to my first wife or my eldest children because they have moved on and are doing their own thing and haven't left a forwarding address or telephone number—I can't say I blame them, the hell I put them all through during my drinking days.

So today for me it's all about not keeping secrets and not behaving badly the way I used to and without going into too many details I was doing things behind my wife's back, not telling her the truth about myself and making excuses about my behaviour usually blaming her for it which was not true at all. I was a very mixed up person long before I ever met her but she was an easy target to blame and it allowed me not to have to look at my part in any of it and not take responsibility for doing something about it. It wasn't until she left that I picked up any responsibility for myself and staggered into AA.

I know this must all sound shocking to you all sitting here but although my behaviour was bad it wasn't motivated by badness. I didn't get up in the mornings and think how can I ruin everyone's life today? I never said to myself I am going to open this bottle and make everybody's life hell. It was always going to be just one drink—but it never worked out like that. I kept doing the same thing over and over again and of course the result was that my family were faced with constant failure too because their hopes were always raised because I might go a couple of days or even weeks without a drink and they would think, this is great he's got it cracked this time and then I would open another bottle and away it would go again. Their hopes were always dashed and it was failure all round really.

The sad thing is when you think this can go on for 10, 20 even 30 years or more, it's no wonder that families get ground down.

The other characteristic is families live in constant hope but those hopes are always dashed. I was living with failure and in a very odd way, in order to compensate for that I became arrogant. So I was putting this publicity around about myself that I was the 'Bees Knees' but inside I knew all of that was rubbish, it was all false but it had become a way of life for me. I was pretending everything was OK but it was far from being OK, it was just a mess really. It was one disaster after another and my mother's life became a mess, my first wife's life became a mess, we ended up just staggering from one disaster to another with hopes that were never fulfilled.

It can be very confusing living with an alcoholic because the 'normal' rules of the game don't apply but the families can't understand that because they are 'normal', well a heck of a lot more 'normal' than the alcoholic is.

It was only when I found my way into AA that I finally got the message and stopped drinking. I have been sober now for over 18 years. Steps 4 & 5 were the beginning of my discovery about who I was. I was able to admit my 'defects of character' as they are called in the AA programme and realise there was nothing so terrible about me, I was just a human being doing the best I could. I no longer had the need to put out this publicity that I was the 'Bees Knees' because actually I wasn't. I was just an OK person doing the best I could and that kind of returned me to 'normality'. So I no longer feel I'm the pits but also I no longer feel I'm Mr Big Shot either because I now know who I am and thank goodness I do.

No wonder people talk about alcoholism being a mental illness because I never knew who I was and not only did I not know but I didn't know that I didn't know! I was just bumbling through life and really hadn't a clue how to handle it at all. It was only by listening to other people's stories that I began to see how life worked and take my place in the scheme of things. I often wonder why someone wasn't able to tell me this 30 years ago because I could have saved myself and my family a heck of a lot of trouble. It's been quite a revelation to find out that actually I'm alright and that was a huge relief because I had laboured all my life thinking I was a terrible person and drinking to cover that up. How sad—it's sad isn't it?

It was all about fear, I was driven by fear, most of my bad behaviour was just me trying to get some fleeting comfort from the ongoing terror and misery I felt all the time. So until I got into recovery and started dealing with my fear nothing was ever going to change for me.

So why was I so full of fear? I really don't know. I had a good childhood—my parents did the best they could. I sort of enjoyed school but looking back I will say I always seemed to have a much more sensitive nervous system than everyone else. I seemed to feel 'the burn' much more than others as if I had a completely different processing system to everyone around me. I couldn't understand any of that at the time—I just knew I perceived the world in a more intense way for some reason.

I think I developed my tough exterior to hide the sensitivity, so I wouldn't be attacked by others around me. So I suppose that's when the hiding and the secrets started and the fear just grew and grew along with that. The only thing I ever found that got rid of my fear was alcohol. When I had a drink I felt released from the burden of having to keep everything repressed and hidden.

Working the 12 Steps has made me feel better about myself because I don't hang on to any negative stuff and I can usually *'Let Go'* of it within a relatively short space of time. Whereas I used to hang on to everything for a long time and let everything fester. Things started to really change for me when I found the courage to do Steps 4 and 5 because before that I didn't look at myself—I just thought well this is who I am and I can't change. But it wasn't true, that wasn't just the way I was going to be forever, I could change.

I think for me finding a HP has helped because I never had much faith and certainly not in myself. In fact, faith in a HP has helped me a great deal to resist the temptation to run away from 'the burn'—so I don't end up behaving badly. I can resist running and hiding from things the way I ran and hid from my alcoholism for years. I ignored it until I couldn't ignore it any longer. I just stuck my head in the sand because I was full of fear of the consequences of what it would mean for me, not for anyone else. I wasn't worried about anyone else. I was worried about what everything meant for me. Yes, I used to pretend and claim to be worried about others, about my wife and kids but really it was all about me being OK and that's the truth of it.

But that's OK today because that's how it was back then in the drinking days and in my early recovery days, it isn't like that today and I hope now that is reflected in how I interact with the world and with people. I hope I'm more fully participating in life in general—I think I am.

In AL, I've learned that a lot of the things I was doing in my relationships were wrong and I had to be prepared to change. So I have found myself setting out on another journey through the same jungle if you like but like I said fortunately I've kind of passed this way before and I know the answers will be in this room and gradually that's been confirmed for me. Both during my years in AA and my time in AL—I have never ever been misguided. It's straightened me out because there were so many things about my thinking that were out of kilter and I think if someone can't afford a psychologist they should join a support group. I didn't know I was all kinked up. I'm just a little bit kinked today, I'm not saying kinky, there is a difference.

Everyone laughs.

But I am gradually getting straightened out and the great thing is, it is giving me serenity and that's what we are promised. We are promised serenity if we accept the things we can't change and have the courage to change the things we can.

Sure, I still have off days when I can feel myself keeling over mentally but I now know when I am keeling over and I go to see my sponsor on a regular basis. I just tell him how I feel and I usually find the problem is caused by me becoming completely occupied with myself. So I have to make a conscious effort to be more concerned about others and I can't do that if I am completely caught up in myself.

I find it's about being honest with myself and knowing who I am. I don't have secrets now and my sponsor knows everything about me. I have no secrets and I want it to be like that because that's how my sponsor can help me. The amount of times I'd thought this pit I had dug for myself was going to be there forever and I was never going to be able to climb out of it because I couldn't see a way out. Then suddenly with a little bit of help it all changes and the message really is in the 12 Steps, it's all here in this programme. All I've got to do is *'Think, Think, Think'* instead of just being on automatic pilot which is what I used to do in the past. Now I *'Think'* and reach out for help to my sponsor and it bears fruit, my problems become solved—I find an option I hadn't seen before.

I'll just finish by saying, I think everybody who has the courage to go to AA has the opportunity of getting sober and everyone who has the courage to come to AL has the opportunity to stay sane because that's what's on offer here—sanity.

And I will just leave it at that thank you."

GROUP TOGETHER

"Thanks Eddie."

KALEB

"Can I come in Alice?

Kaleb's wife is the problem drinker in his life. Kaleb has only been coming to AL for the past few months and although he is in the early

14

stages of recovery, he is already starting to feel the benefits of the group.

Well, for me it took a lot of courage just to come along to this group because I was walking into the unknown but I got to such a point of desperation—I just did it. I suppose I was expecting everyone to be randomly sitting around drinking tea and chatting about how awful it was having alcoholism in their lives. I had no idea there was so much more on offer here, in fact, a whole structure which provides a kind of map for the journey. A map which encourages me to take small steps at my own pace on my own individual journey.

Steps 1, 2 and 3 suggested I trust a HP and this could be anything of my own understanding and since I had no religious faith as such, I decided to put my trust in the group temporarily. I was very wary at first and challenged everything and certainly just chose what I liked and pretty much ignored what I didn't think was useful to me.

I think putting my trust in the group gave me some courage to deal with things because I found it took a lot of pressure off me as I no longer felt I was dealing with everything alone. I felt the wisdom I heard in the group was guiding me so I didn't have to worry so much about getting it completely wrong.

So the help of the group gave me the courage to face a lot of things which I had just ignored and avoided for a long time. For instance, at home I had just ignored unacceptable behaviour that was going on and I think that trait came from my upbringing because I was brought up to believe when you have a problem—you just ignore it. So I think a lot of my problems came from my own unwillingness to talk about things. My alcoholic didn't want to discuss her alcohol problem either so that let me off the hook really but it meant nothing ever got resolved.

So I did find it difficult, well impossible really, to put my cards on the table and have the courage to come out and say what I was thinking and feeling. I wasn't helped by my wife's way of coping with problems—her style is to flare up and shout. Looking back I can see how I lacked the courage to confront her about anything. I had a problem saying don't do that so everything just continued to happen.

When I did my Step 4, I realised a lot of my actions were being driven by fear. I think living with alcoholism had increased my levels of fear to such an extent most of my courage had just gone. I didn't want anything bad to happen to the alcoholic, I didn't want to lose my family. I didn't want to make plans for the future because it all seemed too uncertain.

I think as I have gone through this programme it has provided all of these building blocks which I can use to rebuild my self-esteem which then gives me the courage to start doing some things to help myself to climb out of this hole I was in. I've found once I try something new and it works that gives me more courage to do other things and so gradually it builds up.

So the programme is giving me the strength to be able to change a lot of things. I'm not going to say it's been easy and I'm not going to say it hasn't taken a long time because sometimes it's taken ages just for the penny to drop that something wasn't right. I'm gaining the courage to look at myself and that's a big thing really because I can see the things I have done all of my life and suddenly realise maybe I shouldn't have been doing it like that. Then even more courage is needed to say well maybe I can change that a bit. Without this programme I would have just merrily gone on for the rest of my life doing what I've always done. I get great strength and courage from my fellow members in this room who are always willing to listen and I thank you all for that. Thank you."

GROUP TOGETHER

"Thanks Kaleb."

VICKY

"I'll come in if I may Alice?

16

Vicky spent a couple of years sitting in AA meetings in an attempt to manage her alcoholic daughter's drinking problem. When all her efforts failed a few months ago she finally found her way to an AL meeting.

I think when I first came here it was an act of courage because what I was really saying was I had failed as a mother. I had looked after my daughter all her life, seen her through the teenage years, through the broken romantic relationships, everything—then suddenly the drinking ripped us apart. I felt like a total failure as a mother, almost suicidal. Thankfully once I got here I came to realise I wasn't a failure I'd just done the best I could but because of my ignorance of alcoholism I had done quite a few things wrong. I didn't know I didn't have the power or the knowledge to help her until I came here. Even though we had both worked everything out together up until alcohol entered our lives, I certainly couldn't work alcoholism out. I read every book I could get my hands on but the one thing I would never say was 'I cannot cope' and I think this is the best place ever for me because it helps me to accept I couldn't cope with something as big as this on my own. I didn't really realise before coming here how much courage we have all got to have just to get through life.

Today I can accept that some people cannot cope with the things I can cope with but I also accept that other people can cope with things I can't. I think coming here and admitting I couldn't cure my child, or I was trying to help but didn't have the knowledge to be able to help, was a great act of courage for me.

Also gaining the courage to speak in here, having the courage to be able to talk about very tough times in my life and share my experiences so others may benefit from them too has been tough for me.

Oh and I found it wasn't only my daughter's drinking bouts I had to deal with I also had the ripple effects it had on the rest of the family to cope with. My husband and I deal with things in completely different ways and he gets angry and puts his blinkers on and I found I used to really dread the binges because of what it did to her but also because

I knew what was coming—from him. So even though she doesn't live with us now her alcoholism is still causing all of this bother in the house. Just recently I found the courage to tackle him about his outbursts because I had just had enough. I used the programme and a cup of coffee to deliver my message in a calm and gentle manner. I said 'you know your angry outbursts give me more heartache than our daughter when she is drinking' and he couldn't believe what I was saying. But he must have thought about it because something changed and he doesn't disagree with me seeing her now while she is on one of her binges. So that was definitely the programme and talking to fellow members and being able to explain things in such a way and not get angry so I was able to get through to him and he hasn't had the same angry outbursts since. So that is one example of practising the programme that took courage for me to do because it used to be like lighting a fuse paper with him at times and that's obviously how he copes with it and its quite sad really because we have been together for years and he is a wonderful husband but alcoholism is so powerful it can come between anything. And that's all I've got to say at the moment, thank you."

GROUP TOGETHER

"Thanks Vicky."

CLARISSA

"Can I come in Alice?

Clarissa is a woman in her mid-30's who is married to an alcoholic. He had 2 years of sobriety but has occasionally picked up again over the past 6 months.

I found it very hard to come along to this meeting for the first time and I remember being physically sick in the car park before I came in, that's how much fear I felt and how much courage I needed to feel the fear and do it anyway.

Then when I got in and sat listening to everyone I heard people saying they had been doing things wrong and the word wrong just triggered negative feelings in me because I didn't want to hear that I had been doing things wrong because my self-esteem was already on the floor because the alcoholic had told me for years that everything I did was wrong. So I had to find the courage to try new things. So even if I find myself shaking the first time I try something, I find it's not so bad when I do it again. For me it's repeating it because if I get the courage to do something once I can repeat it and do it again. All I have to do is keep on going until I get so used to it—it becomes second nature to me. I still find it difficult with certain things, I can get frightened and I need the courage to deal with things on a daily basis so I do *One day at a Time* and if I am really in trouble I get on the phone and just say I'm struggling here I need an AL chat. I agree with what people have said tonight it does take courage to admit we need help. It even took courage to admit to myself I needed help and I wasn't coping. I certainly didn't cope with the alcoholism, I thought I did but I made some big, big mistakes because I had no idea what would help. I think the 12 Step programme should be on the National Curriculum to help kids to cope with life, it certainly would have helped me to make some better choices if I had learned this years ago.

And I'll just leave it there, Thanks."

GROUP TOGETHER

"Thanks Clarissa."

MACK

"Can I come in Alice?

Mack is a regular at AL meetings. He is a man of around 60 and comes from a family of Irish descent. He retired on grounds of ill-health at 52, which he believes is the result of obsessively trying to stop his alcoholic son from drinking.

As we all know alcoholism spreads across families and I came here obsessed with my son's—well obsessed with my son, full stop. I thought I could fix him which I tried for some time then I came here and listened and learned and I'm sitting here tonight NOT obsessed with my son, so that for me is a result.

I'm glad I'm here tonight and have you all to listen to. Thank you."

GROUP TOGETHER

"Thanks Mack."

PIPPA

"I'll just briefly share Alice.

Pippa's boyfriend is the drinker in her life. She came along to the group some time ago but left after a few meetings. She is back because of a current crisis she needs support with.

This week I've cried and cried, I think it takes courage to cry.

Pippa pauses and starts crying before continuing.

Look I'm doing it again! I think it takes courage to honour my feelings and not just stuff them away and hide them to make others feel more comfortable. I think it's a weakness not to be able to cry. It's not self-pity, it's sadness, I'm sad the person I love most in the world is killing himself with alcohol. I suppose this is me trying to have the courage to accept that I'm not in control of all of this and I need to keep coming here for your support.

Thank you."

GROUP TOGETHER

"Thanks Pippa."

ALICE

"I'm mindful of the time but we do have about 7 minutes left if anyone who hasn't already spoken would like to come in and share?"

STAVROS

"I will just quickly come in Alice?

The alcoholic in Stavros' life was his wife. He does not know whether she is still alive or not. The last time he heard any news of her, she was spotted living on the streets but he has never been able to track her down.

When I came here it was suggested I could help myself by trying to practice the 12 Steps. I suppose it took courage to keep coming back and be willing to look at myself. I've discovered so many things about myself that I would never have known. I've discovered shortcomings which I was blind to but I've also unearthed so many good points I was equally blind to, so it has been a real learning curve for me. I feel I've come a long way in working out who I am and have learned some very good coping strategies into the bargain. I feel it is all pretty healthy stuff and it has brought me so much peace of mind and that's all I'd like to say, thank you."

GROUP TOGETHER

"Thanks Stavros."

MACK

"I'll come in Alice."

ALICE

"Thanks Mack."

MACK

"Thanks everyone for your shares. If I had to choose one useful thing I can take home with me tonight from this meeting it's the acknowledgment that 'I can't choose the cards'. Life happens and we are just left having to find the courage to deal with whatever comes our way. I've seen amazing acts of courage in this room over the time I've been a member and that has given me strength to go forward myself and live my own life to the very best of my ability.

Thanks everyone."

GROUP TOGETHER

"Thanks Mack."

ALICE

"So it's that time again so can I just remind our recent members we suggest you come back for at least 6 meetings before you decide whether it's for you or not. The reason we say that is because we have different members and different topics here at different times and it could be that you don't find anyone you feel you can identify with at your first few meetings.

However, if after 6 meetings you find no identification then the group is probably either not for you or not for you at this time.

Before we close our meeting tonight I will just remind everybody of the theme for next time is—

One Day at a Time

Do we have a volunteer to be the main sharer for next time?"

There is a long pause.

KALEB

"I will be the main sharer next time, Alice."

ALICE

"Thank You Kaleb.

So it just remains for me to say that there are no dues for membership but we do ask you to make a contribution of whatever you can afford to cover our costs for tea and coffee and rent. If you cannot afford anything then that is OK too.

OK, I'm afraid our time is up and we close on time, so Mack, can I ask you to read the suggested closing to close our meeting please?"

MACK

"In closing, I would like to say that the opinions expressed here were strictly those of the person who gave them. Take what you liked and leave the rest. A few words to those of you who haven't been with us long: whatever your problems, there are those amongst us who have had them too. If you try to keep an open mind, you will find help. You will come to realise that there is no situation too difficult to be bettered and no unhappiness too great to be lessened.

Will all those who care to join me in closing our meeting?"

Everyone joins hands in a circle.

GROUP TOGETHER

"Grant me the Serenity to accept the things I cannot change.
The courage to change the things I can and
The wisdom to know the difference.
Same time, Same Place, Keep coming back, it works if you work it."

Meeting 5

Tonight's Topic—One Day at a Time

AL stands for Alcoholics' Loved Ones and is a meeting for anyone who is, or has been, affected by someone else's drinking, regardless of whether the person is still drinking or not.

STAVROS says,

"Ok, shall we make a start everybody?

One of the disciplines in AL is we start on time and we finish on time, regardless.

So, I will read the suggested opening:

We would like to welcome you to this AL meeting.

The AL meeting is a group of relatives and friends of problem drinkers who share their experience, strength and hope in order to solve their common problems. We believe alcoholism is a family illness and that changed attitudes can aid recovery.

Although we have no newcomers here tonight, I would still like us to go round the room and introduce ourselves, using first names only because it takes us all a little time to remember everybody's name."

Meet the Group

STAVROS

"I'm Stavros and I'm chairing the meeting tonight. It was my wife who was dependent on alcohol and trying to live with the impact that had on my own life brought me into this group."

CLARISSA

"Hello, I'm Clarissa and the alcoholic in my life is my husband but I am here tonight for me."

VICKY

"Hello, I'm Vicky and the problem drinker in my life is my daughter."

EDDIE

"I'm Eddie and as most of you know I'm a 'double-winner'. That simply means I'm a member of two support groups. I'm a recovering alcoholic but I'm also married to a recovering alcoholic so I qualify for membership of AL too as I have a family member who is an alcoholic."

JOSH

"Hello, my name's Josh and as you all know, I'm quite new to the group."

JEFF

"My name is Jeff and the person with the drink problem in our life is our son. My wife Alice is here tonight with me. Our son is still drinking heavily and is drunk most days."

INGRID

"I'm Ingrid and I'm fairly new to the group but I have already started to feel much better since coming here."

PIPPA

"Hello, I'm Pippa and I am back tonight because I desperately need the support I can get from the group."

MACK

"Hi, I'm Mack and it's my son who is addicted to alcohol".

ELSA

"Hello I'm Elsa and I've been coming to AL for 8 years and it is my father who is the alcoholic in my life."

ALICE

"Hello, my name is Alice and as Jeff said earlier it is our son who has a problem with alcohol."

KALEB

"Hello, I'm Kaleb and I'm really glad to be here tonight."

*   *   *

STAVROS

"Can I remind everyone that this is an anonymous group and we use first names only. Anonymity is one of the key principles we adhere to in the group.

You do not need to tell us who you are, where you live, where you work, what you do—absolutely nothing about your personal details at all if you don't want to.

There are 12 of us here tonight but the numbers vary each week and sometimes there are more of us and sometimes less.

You don't have to come every week but we do suggest you attend as regularly as you can if you want to benefit from what's on offer here. Our only purpose is to share our experience, strength and hope to help ourselves and each other to gain some peace of mind because our lives have been affected by an alcohol dependent person. Anything else about your life is no concern of ours unless you choose to share it with us.

So, as I've said my name is Stavros and although I am chairing the meeting tonight, next time someone else will be chairing because we practice the principle of rotation of leadership in the group.

A special word for our recent members, it may all still seem strange and you will probably go away not understanding much about what you hear tonight but if you feel something that brings you back then that is enough to be going on with. Just keep coming back and it will eventually start to become much clearer about what support you can gain from the group.

Also, although we meet up in a church hall this programme is not religious and has no connection to any church. The only reason we meet here is because of low costs.

So on with the meeting. Every week we have a different theme and tonight's theme is:

One Day at a Time

Jeff can you start us off with the 12 steps please?"

JEFF

"Step 1: We admitted we were powerless over the problem drinker and that our lives had become unmanageable."

INGRID

"Step 2: We came to believe that a power greater than ourselves could restore us to serenity."

PIPPA

"Step 3: We made a decision to turn our will and our lives over to the care of our higher power (HP)."

MACK

"Step 4: We made a searching and fearless moral inventory of ourselves."

ELSA

"Step 5: We admitted to our HP, to ourselves and to another human being the exact nature of our wrongs."

ALICE

"Step 6: We were entirely ready to have our HP remove all these defects of character."

KALEB

"Step 7: We humbly asked our HP to remove our shortcomings."

STAVROS

"Step 8: We made a list of all persons we had harmed and became willing to make amends to them all."

CLARISSA

"Step 9: We made direct amends to such people wherever possible, except when to do so would injure them or others."

VICKY

"Step 10: We continued to take personal inventory and when we were wrong promptly admitted it."

EDDIE

"Step 11: We sought through reflection and meditation to improve our conscious contact with our HP, seeking only knowledge of our HP's will for us and the power to carry that out."

JOSH

"Step 12: Having had an emotional and spiritual awakening as the result of these Steps, we tried to carry this message to others, and to practice these principles in all our affairs."

*   *   *

STAVROS

"Kaleb has agreed to be our main sharer for tonight and can I just remind you there is no obligation for anyone to share. You can remain silent and just listen if you prefer but those who do decide to share are allowed to do so without interruption from others. So over to you Kaleb, on the theme of—**One Day at a Time.**"

KALEB

"Thanks everyone for being here tonight.

Kaleb's wife is the alcoholic in his life. She regularly tries to give up drinking herself without any help from support services. Sometimes she goes for months without drinking but so far has always started again. She continues to deny she has a problem with alcohol.

Living *'One Day at a Time'* is something I have had to learn and I now find it extremely useful. For instance, I had a presentation to give at work the other day and in the past I would have worried about it all night and rushed into work early to try to sort out any last minute problems. I would have been very anxious about it all. However, now I don't do any of that. My behaviour has changed remarkably because I just think I can deal with that tomorrow and

I don't need to think about it today. I just *'Let it Go'* and live in the now. So I do see this as a skill which I have learned and which I have to put into practice to get the results I want. My main goal is always—peace of mind. In fact, sometimes I practice telling myself I only have to live in the hour, or I only have to live in the minute if I am experiencing a lot of stress.

I used to project manage everything and had giant lists that I was never going to get through. I've stopped all of that now. Leaving yesterday behind I think is something I have dealt with to a large extent in Step 4. One shortcoming I had was I used to keep going back over events saying 'what if' I'd done that differently? I used to drive myself nuts. It was just a recipe for self-dissatisfaction. I've stopped all of that now, I really have and again that's all come about by my practising this principle of *'One day at a Time'*. For me it's about looking back but not staring back and getting obsessed about things that did or didn't happen.

Before coming into AL I had very poor coping strategies for dealing with stress. Now my belief is if I do my best today then tomorrow is likely to be as good as it can be. So I think that is an interesting lesson I have learned.

I have also had lots of difficulties with my children because of how they have been affected by living with alcoholism. They haven't necessarily done things the way I thought they should have done them. Now they are 20 and 18 and I could have worried about them quite a lot. I am certainly concerned about them from time to time but I try not to worry about them because I do believe in them and I have faith in them that they will get to where they need to be. I think I was unwittingly robbing them of their own self-confidence by always trying to micro-manage them in the direction of doing things which felt comfortable for me.

I think it's interesting how my son dropped out of his college course because he didn't like doing it and there was far too much going on at home for him to focus on studying. I was annoyed about his decision at first but then I decided I just had to accept it was his call and not mine. It is his life so he knows much more than me what he can cope with at this time.

Dropping out of college is something I would never have dreamed of doing when I was his age—I would have just battled on to the bitter end. He feels it's a learning process and he wants to start again next year doing totally different subjects. At one time I would have been in there trying to force solutions to fit in with my perspective on life but now I don't think that's my job. He's got to decide what he is going to do next—he's got to work that out for himself. That's all part and parcel of him growing-up.

So I do care for him but I try to keep the focus on myself and not worry about him because I have to have faith he can work it out for himself. If he needs my help he will ask for it without me storming in and trying to 'run the show' in my own image so to speak. I try to give him as much advice as I can but when I start getting the Oh! 'in the olden days' comments I know it is well time for me to back off and leave him to it. There is only so much he will take before the shutters go up and I am frozen out if I just continue to bang my drum at him.

Yes, it is difficult not to get involved but when their mother gets involved she just jumps up and down shouting and screaming at them, until a big conflict breaks out, so I think if I stay calm they will stay calm and not get caught up in the madness of it all. I say to my kids, look don't do anything without first calming down and discussing it at length, talk it through about how you are feeling and about why you want to do this. I do manage to stay in the day and live one day at a time, most of the time but not always, I'm still working on it. Thank You."

GROUP TOGETHER

"Thanks Kaleb."

EDDIE

"I will come in here Stavros?

Eddie is both a recovering alcoholic himself (sober for over 18 years) and a member of AL because he is married to Sarah who is also a recovering alcoholic.

Ok, well where should I start with this one?

I suppose I can share how it was for me before I found the group. I used to be terrible for living in the past and then worrying myself to death about what was going to happen in the future. My head just wouldn't stop. I used to go around picking up loads of resentments about people and nurturing my anger about them and then dragging them along with me through my life. My own resentments used to eat me alive. It was that kind of thinking which led to me pouring the booze down my neck so I could blot out the constant negative chattering that was going around in my head.

That kind of thinking doesn't happen for me now because I have done everything the programme has suggested and it's worked for me. Yes, things can still get to me because I am only human but I now recognise very quickly what's going on inside of me and I stop and make a conscious decision about which tool of the programme I am going to apply to any given event.

I am all for living in the day now and I think the *'One Day at a Time'* slogan is a brilliant one for me to use because common sense tells me I cannot do anything about the past, it's gone. Yes, I can remember events or incidents and use them as kind of reference points and guidelines for today, in that, I suppose I can learn from my mistakes if I remember when I did A, then the consequences of B, happened and that caused a negative outcome. I heard it said in AA, don't close the door on the past because it is an asset and I can learn valuable lessons from it but at the same time I cannot sit around and agonise about what I should have done or could have done because I can't go back and undo it.

I have learned if I stay resentful about things in my past they will just stick around and haunt me. I have learned this from very bitter experience. For a long time I used to carry around negative past events and nurtured them until they grew and grew to the point where they consumed me. I can remember thinking I can't go on living like this because I just kept constantly mulling over things and they distracted me from the useful things I could have been getting on with today.

Slowly, with the help of the programme I have been able to put a lot of these ghosts to rest. I realised the 'if-only's' were absolutely pointless and it was only then that I started to *Let Go* of them. So all of those years when I nurtured and clung on to my resentments who did I actually hurt by it? Me! So the lesson I have learned is it doesn't matter about the past there is nothing I can do about it now.

The reason I am constantly practicing the skill of living in the day is because it gives me peace of mind and I find that is vital to me if I am going to do anything constructive and useful today. If I am not alright in my head then nothing's right and I don't want to go back to that place because that is what started me off drinking all those years ago. I have been in AA for quite a long time and I came to understand that drinking was not my first problem, my first problem was my thinking and I used to drink to escape from the intolerable mental turmoil that I lived in all the time. As soon as the alcoholic is separated from the booze all of that thinking is still there and my real job in AA was to sort out my thinking.

I think a lot of addiction is down to habit and this also applies to the alcoholics family members because they just keep doing what they have always done even though it doesn't work. The family keep trying to force solutions without being fully aware of what they are doing.

Coming to the group has prompted me to ask myself why I do certain things. I question myself now as to whether or not I should be doing a certain thing, just because I have always done it that way, doesn't mean to say its right. I had always done what I had always done and

I came here and suddenly realised that some of my behaviour was not acceptable and I have been prompted to take steps to change it.

As for my future, I'm a list person now, I didn't used to be but now I've got myself a bit more organised with the help of the programme. I make myself lists and I do exactly what I need to do, the aim is at the end of the day to have everything crossed off and finished. The theory is great but it didn't work first time around because I was finding I had masses of stuff still on my list at the end of the day until I realised I was setting myself impossible goals with great lists of things and if I stood back and looked at them I could see I was never going to get through them all.

So what I try to do now is, I set myself a small number of realisable goals and clearly some things I have to have at the top of the list because they are very important. The problem I have is that things occur during the day and they leap to the top of my list because they have to be done so it is rare if I can get to the end of the day and my list is cleared off. But I can be kind to myself today and not beat myself up about it. I can say look there are a couple of things I haven't got done but really does it matter anyway, not really, so I put them on my list for tomorrow and in all probability they could go to the bottom again and remain undone as well but—so what!

This is all part of the manageability that's been restored to me by working the 12 steps and looking sensibly at what needs to be done, concentrating on it, and doing it. I know when I get it right because I get that nice satisfying feeling at the end of the day that I might have done a few important things and got them out of the way. That is a huge difference to how I used to do things, I used to get to the end of the day and be filled with trepidation and anxiety, having panicked all day because I wasn't getting all of these things done and at the end of it all none of them actually got done because I'd do a bit of that one and move on and did a bit of another one and at the end of it all none of it was actually done properly so I felt like a failure because I had achieved nothing, whereas now, because I suppose I am being more realistic and more disciplined I find I achieve more.

I would say I am quite good at this now, leaving yesterday behind. In my drinking days I heard people say funny things in AA and sometimes, expressed a bit graphically, but they were usually very true, I heard someone say ' . . . if you've got one foot in yesterday and one foot in tomorrow you are just pissing on today . . .' And that is how I used to live because I was always pissing on today, thinking if only I had done something differently. Looking back I realise I had lived like that for such a long time and just because I stopped drinking didn't mean I stopped all of these self-sabotaging behaviour patterns I had learned along the way. It took real hard work and discipline to get those changed.

Now when I get up in the morning yesterday has gone. It's finished with. Tomorrow is another matter I can make plans and that is part of my making a list. I don't think any human being can live their life without planning stuff even if it's just when to pay the bills and where to go on holiday. I think they are normal things. I make a list and I think well whatever ends up on this list undone can go back on the list tomorrow because I have got enough on my plate getting myself through today.

It was part of my alcoholic thinking to think life ought to be all 'plain sailing', without any problems and it took me a long time to realise how ridiculous that belief was because life is often hard work and sometimes it is not very nice.

However today, I am pleased to say most of the time I have peace of mind and my 'racing brain' is kept well and truly in check by working this programme. I try my best to keep everything in the day and I don't constantly worry about things and when my head reaches the pillow at night I sleep like a baby and it's wonderful.

I would describe my life now as a gentle rollercoaster ride sometimes it is happy and exciting other times it's quiet—just getting on with things and if I can keep my life disciplined like that then I'm doing OK. One thing that will definitely perturb my gentle rollercoaster ride will be bringing in regrets from yesterday and then importing fears from tomorrow. I really just do what it says there

Eddie points to the card on the table with the slogan 'One Day at a Time' on it.

I live *'One Day at a Time'* and for me it is just a great formula and the beauty of it is—it's simple and that's what I like. Thanks everyone."

GROUP TOGETHER

"Thanks Eddie."

INGRID

"I will come in here Stavros.

Ingrid is a newcomer to AL. Her husband is a binge drinker so she never knows when he is going to start drinking again. She lives in constant fear of his drinking bouts and her own physical and mental health are being affected by it.

Thanks Kaleb & Eddie for your shares and thanks everybody for being here.

Eddie—you have clarified it for me where my own issues lie with regards to living *'One day at a time'*. I don't think I have a lot of problems with leaving yesterday behind because I find I am constantly anticipating what awful things might happen tomorrow. The only time I look back at the past is perhaps when I am feeling tired or out of sorts and then sometimes I can start feeling sorry for myself and think Oh Poor Me! But most of the time I never have the time to think of the past my mind is so focussed on what lies ahead.

In fact I think this is my biggest problem, having a mind which races ahead and thinks about what lies down the road for me and that stops me from enjoying today. I'm always saying to myself—Oh no! What is going to happen next? It's always a kind of dread. When I first joined the group my husband was in the middle of one of his binges but now he is OK'ish but I am still thinking no one can live like this and he's going to die very soon. So I'm thinking oh I can't stay here and I began to make plans to move away. Now when I look at my life, it is all very different. He is not drinking and I have made some recovery myself. So from experience I should feel that I don't know what is going to happen and life is full of pleasant surprises too and I am immensely grateful for the blessings I do have in my life and one of them is this group.

I don't know whether 'living in the day' is a skill or an art and it sounds so simple but it can be so hard to do because my head just runs away with me. For instance, when my daughter happens to make some comment on how alcoholism has impacted badly on her life I immediately think 'bad mother' I should have done things differently, I should have left the alcoholic years ago, I should have done this and I should have done that but then the programme kicks in and I can remind myself to back off, take the pressure off myself and stop beating myself up because you know what—I did the best I could at the time. That was my best. It might not have been good enough but it was my very best and I can't expect any more than that from myself. It was the best I could do given my own thinking and experience I had at that time.

I think being in a 'battle' is a very good description of how it feels to live with alcoholism. I've noticed people in the room often use this word when they are describing the energy around living with the alcoholic. I certainly felt as if I was using all of my resources just to keep things going and keep things manageable around the alcoholic. So when I start to use the programme and find myself no longer in 'battle' mode, those battling habits I have obviously become accustomed to are very difficult to get rid of. I feel like I am one of those old-fashioned lorries which takes so, so much time to grind to a stop before being able to turn everything around.

This also reminds me of a trip I had to the Australian outback years ago when I visited some small isolated villages where everyone just lived in the day. The experience left a big impression on me because they just 'were'. I was amazed at the sharp contrast with our culture where we are all brought up to believe we should be achieving all the time. We have to be doing things all the time otherwise we feel guilty in some way. OK I'm not suggesting we all live like Australian bush people but I do think we can have more of a balance between 'always doing' and 'just being' and I think the imbalance is getting even worse as our culture speeds up to keep pace with technology. I ask myself should we be aligning ourselves with machines that don't have a need for balance the way we do, is it healthy for us? From where I am sitting I would say absolutely not, it's a fool's gold.

But my mind does just run riot about what is going to happen next so the problem for me is tomorrow, I have got to stop trying to take on tomorrow all the time and thank god I've got AL to help me do it."

GROUP TOGETHER

"Thanks Ingrid."

After a long pause where everyone seems deep in thought . . .

STAVROS

"Would anyone else like to come in?"

PIPPA

"I will come in, if I may Stavros?

Pippa attended AL for 3 meetings last year but decided it wasn't for her. She came back recently because of a current crisis she feels she needs support with.

I don't normally sit down for very long but I was sitting down today thinking about what I was going to say on this topic tonight. I have felt sad for weeks. I think as my life is changing—I think I was just in a habit because I was living with the alcoholic and I lived in the moment expecting x, y and z to happen and the more times I went through the alcoholism, I adapted my behaviour, by trying this and if that didn't work I would try something else and—nothing ever worked. So really I was just working around the alcoholic. I didn't feel as if I had any choices, even though I know now I did always have choices—I just couldn't see them at the time. I was thinking 'oh if I tried something else I might be able to fix it next time' and I didn't.

And it's strange when I sit down and think I've been willing to change everything about my own behaviour to try to keep him happy but all of those changes haven't been the correct changes and therefore in reality nothing has changed much for the better. My method was wrong, the tools I was using were wrong and so all of that effort has amounted to absolutely zero.

And I think that is why I get angry with myself for not seeking help sooner. I just battled on alone thinking I could sort it all out. I used to get frustrated with myself for not changing quickly enough and not anticipating quickly enough what would keep him happy. When really almost everything I was doing was wrong.

I think what I had been doing was when he came out of his drunken states of oblivion I spent a lot of my time trying to remember all the things I wanted to say to him that I couldn't say to him while he was drunk. I didn't get to say things when he was out of it. So all the arguments and all the different things I wanted to say to him I stored up and waited to pounce when he had sobered up. I wanted to say I was right and he was wrong. I had a great need to be right. But after all the arguing I was no further forward and I ended up just letting him think he was right when he wasn't so we could get back to living this egg-shell walking life-style we had going on.

It was great when we were having a good day but when we had a bad day I could forget about it very quickly. I don't know whether it was because I had experienced so many rough times that I just wanted to grab those good days and hold on to them to get me through the awful times.

It's taken me a long time to even realise what I have been doing. I have just been on automatic pilot most of the time and reacting to his provocations instead of seeking the help I needed from others who have walked this path before me. I am very pleased to be here tonight to listen to all of your shares. Thank you."

GROUP TOGETHER

"Thanks Pippa."

ALICE

"I wasn't going to come in but I think I should because I've had a really bad week and I need to get back on track.

Alice comes to the group with her husband Jeff. It is their son who has an alcohol addiction.

Speaking of 'yesterdays'—well I had a bad beginning to the week. It was Mother's Day on Sunday which was a bad day because I didn't hear from my son. I started off well on the Sunday morning. I thought well I'm really strong here today then everything went pear shaped in the afternoon. I just flipped and let rip at my husband. Monday wasn't much better I just didn't want to speak to anybody I wanted to be left on my own. My mind was working overtime and I've never felt the way I did these last 2 days. Both Sunday and Monday I was just totally wound up inside, totally angry with everything, I just couldn't get my head around things. The phone was ringing and I knew it was my friend phoning for a chat but I wouldn't answer the phone, I just let it ring and ring. I thought no I don't want to speak to anybody. Then I thought I'd better ring her back and tell her I don't want to speak because I know she is going through some tough times herself at the moment but I didn't feel like I could be a very good friend this week. So I phoned and told her I just wanted to be on my own and didn't want to speak this week.

Eventually, I thought I have got to try and sort this out and get my head around things and get back to working the programme. But I've never felt like that inside before, I was just wild with anger. I felt dreadful. I was just thinking daft things in my head, was he drunk somewhere, had he been killed in a car accident, all that daft stuff just kept coming in and sending my head racing from one catastrophe to another. I was also thinking there are some really nasty people in the world so why has this curse of alcoholism had to happen to my son? I'm trying to get strong again now. Today hasn't been so bad I'm feeling a bit better today but I think I have got to get back to taking just *'One day at a time'* again. And I will just leave it at that."

GROUP TOGETHER

"Thanks Alice."

JEFF

"I'll just follow on from Alice if I can Stavros.

Jeff is married to Alice and it is their son who is dependent on alcohol.

I know Alice has been very upset this week with our son's recent disappearing act, especially since it was Mother's day last Sunday but I have come to expect this from him and I have been practising the slogan *'Live and Let Live'*. It's his choice and I try to stick to the philosophy of living in the day and let him get on and do whatever he is going to do. That's all I want to say thanks."

GROUP TOGETHER

"Thanks Jeff."

CLARISSA

"I'll come in Stavros.

Clarissa's husband is the alcoholic in her life and has suffered from mental health problems related to his drinking. He has tried several

41

alcohol recovery groups but still has 'slips'. He is currently not drinking.

I think that's what's great about this programme—we only have to concentrate on *'One day at a time'*. For instance, when my husband picked up the drink again after being sober for over 2 years and whilst in a drunken stupor tried to commit suicide—I was utterly, utterly devastated. I remember thinking I really, really know now what the 'end of your tether' means because I have reached it.

I was like a spaced out zombie for days. I was just wandering around in a daze, just shock, despair—I was at the absolute end of my tether. So what got me through it? I can remember thinking I will just do what I would normally be doing. I would get the clothes ready for the next day. I would make the school lunch-boxes and put them in the hall the night before. I had three kids to see to so I decided to behave as normally as possible until I got through this crisis.

When all this happened I had been in AL for over a year and I found if I stuck as strictly as I possibly could to the programme I could get through it. Yes, I dipped very badly for over a week but I was amazed at how quickly I came back up. Some of my family members thought I was coming back up so quickly because my husband was getting better in hospital but I knew the truth, it had nothing to do with him. I was bouncing back quickly because I was being so strict with myself in following this programme and that's what pulled me through.

So I pretty much know from experience that if it happened again or any crisis for that matter, I would probably dip again but it is not how low I would fall it's how quickly I would bounce back that makes me realise whether I am working the programme or not because although for a week after I was in a total daze and don't know how I functioned, I did very soon pull through but if I hadn't of had the programme I wouldn't have got better because I wouldn't have known what to do and that's why I think really getting into the programme and shutting out all other thoughts and just concentrating on getting through *'One day at a time'*, sometimes 10 minutes at a time was what did it for me. I felt much better because of it. Looking back on it now I can see that I was able to be my own best friend and act in my own interests. I also had the meetings and my AL friends to support me and I can't tell you how grateful I am for that. Thank you."

GROUP TOGETHER

"Thanks Clarissa."

ELSA

"I will come in Stavros.

Elsa is a long-time member of the group. She is the adult child of an alcoholic father (ACOA). Her father has been a sober alcoholic for 25 years in AA.

I haven't thought about this topic at all for tonight but sometimes I think that is a good thing because then it comes straight from the heart and not my head. When I came here years ago I felt like I was in the right place. I felt like I had been wrapped up in a nice warm blanket because the people who were sharing that night were talking about how I felt inside and I hadn't heard anybody talk about their feelings for years and years. Having an alcoholic father created so much mayhem in our house when I was growing up that I felt I missed out on a lot of the nurturing and caring that most children get. It was only when I came here that I heard people describing my feelings which I couldn't even describe for myself at that time. I just knew I wasn't happy but I didn't have a clue why not. I didn't realise in my case it was fear, resentment and pain and all that other stuff I couldn't have named. I couldn't name all of the pain that was stored up inside of me but gradually I did learn in AL how to name a feeling when it rose up from my feet so to speak. Then I started to feel better than I had done in a long time.

I practised a lot of the stuff which was suggested in here and it helped me to feel better about myself. The foundational tool for me was *'One Day at a Time'* because I found I could achieve more by living in the day, in fact, as some people have already shared tonight, it can be an hour or even a minute at a time, when things get really rough.

So I don't give myself a hard time anymore trying to be perfect, trying to keep everybody happy, I've started to accept myself as I am. The twists and turns of my personal development in AL have certainly given me some steep learning curves at times. I now see this programme as a continuous circle of learning and it is suggested that we do it *'One Day at a Time'* because that's how it works best and I have experienced that to be the case.

I think that's about as much as I want to say tonight. Thank you."

<u>GROUP TOGETHER</u>

"Thanks Elsa."

<u>VICKY</u>

"Can I come in Stavros?

Vicky's daughter has a problem with alcohol.

I think I am OK with leaving yesterday behind—my problem is obsessing about the future. I am constantly trying to stop the 'what-ifs' and although I say I can leave yesterday behind I do remember all the bad times, I have no malice about them but they are still there at the back of my mind all the horror that was happening and how bad it was. The stuff I was going through and the fear of that happening again and I can't no matter how much I've tried, stop that.

I could be feeling great one minute and then for no reason I find myself looking for signs, for instance, when she doesn't arrive when she says she will, or when she seems to be getting more irritable than usual, I'm fearful and I am looking all the time for little signs to warn me because I have seen signs in the past which did in fact lead to her drinking again.

So something will just trigger me off and then it is on my mind, it's the fear and I think 'Oh what is going to happen here?' and then I try and remember AL and everyone in the group and I talk to myself and calm myself down and it does help me but it doesn't stop me having these fears which come back time and time again. So although I am learning to cope a lot better I still find it very hard to stay in the day and not jump into the middle of next week or next year. Thanks."

GROUP TOGETHER

"Thanks Vicky."

Stavros keeps an eye on the time.

STAVROS

"Well we have about 3 or 4 minutes left of the meeting if anyone would like to come in with a short share or two very short shares."

JOSH

"I will come in Stavros.

Josh is a medical student. The drinker in his life was his twin sister who died a year ago.

I still feel very new to the group but one thing I do know is I need to find peace in my life and I do feel a big measure of peace just sitting in this room listening to you all, so I suppose that is a very good start for me. People say things and I go home and mull over them and some of it starts to make sense.

Tonight I have realised that I do live in the day at work because the type of job I have sort of demands it but once I take my work hat off and go home it's a totally different story. I start dwelling on a whole chain of regrets from the past, mostly to do with my sister. I blame myself for not doing more to help her but I had no idea what to do. I tried so many different things and nothing made any difference so I suppose I just turned to humiliation and criticism to try to control her behaviour and try to get her to drink less. I suppose I sat in judgement of her and didn't behave very kindly because of it.

I now feel very ashamed and regretful about that but as Eddie said there is nothing I can do about the past now, it's gone and I'm only torturing myself by not accepting that. I think I have an awful lot to learn about the acceptance of another perception. As for '*One day at a Time*', I suppose I will have to do it before I will know whether it works for me or not. I think if I am ever going to find some peace in this situation it is going to be with the help of you all in here. Thank you."

GROUP TOGETHER

"Thanks Josh."

STAVROS

"Can I just remind our recent members that we suggest you come back for at least 6 meetings before you decide whether it's for you or not. The reason we say that is because we have different members and different topics here at different times and it could be that you don't find anyone you feel you can identify with at your first few meetings. However, if after 6 meetings you find no identification then the group is probably either not for you or not for you at this time.

Before we close our meeting tonight I will just remind everybody of the theme for next time is—

Looking for Help

Do we have a volunteer to be the main sharer for next time?"

MACK

"I will be the main sharer Stavros."

STAVROS

"Thank You, Mack.

So it just remains for me to say that there are no dues for membership but we do ask you to make a contribution of whatever you can afford to cover our costs for tea and coffee and rent. If you cannot afford anything then that is OK too.

OK, I'm afraid our time is up and we close on time, so Kaleb, can I ask you to read the suggested closing to close our meeting please?"

KALEB

"In closing, I would like to say that the opinions expressed here were strictly those of the person who gave them. Take what you liked and leave the rest. A few words to those of you who haven't been with us long: whatever your problems, there are those amongst us who have had them too. If you try to keep an open mind, you will find help. You will come to realise that there is no situation too difficult to be bettered and no unhappiness too great to be lessened.

Will all those who care to join me in closing our meeting?"

Everyone joins hands in a circle

GROUP TOGETHER

"Grant me the Serenity to accept the things I cannot change.
The courage to change the things I can and
The wisdom to know the difference.
Same time, Same Place, Keep coming back, it works if you work it."

Meeting 6

Tonight's Topic—Looking for Help?

AL stands for Alcoholics' Loved Ones and is a meeting for anyone who is, or has been, affected by someone else's drinking, regardless of whether the person is still drinking or not.

EDDIE says,

"Ok everybody, shall we make a start"?

One of the disciplines in AL is we start on time and we finish on time, regardless.

So, I will read the suggested opening:

We would like to welcome you to this AL meeting.

The AL meeting is a group of relatives and friends of problem drinkers who share their experience, strength and hope in order to solve their common problems. We believe alcoholism is a family illness and that changed attitudes can aid recovery.

I would like to welcome you to this AL meeting and although we have no newcomers here tonight I would still like us to go round the room and introduce ourselves, using first names only because it takes us all a little time to remember everybody's name."

Meet the Group

EDDIE

"I'm Eddie and I'm chairing the meeting tonight. As most of you know I'm a 'double-winner' which simply means I'm a member of two support groups. I'm a recovering alcoholic myself and I'm also married to a recovering alcoholic so I qualify for membership of AL too as I have a family member who is alcohol dependent."

STAVROS

"I'm Stavros and it was my ex-wife who was the drinker in my life and trying to live with the impact that had on my own life brought me into this group."

CLARISSA

"Hello, I'm Clarissa and the alcoholic in my life is my husband but I am here tonight for me."

VICKY

"Hello, I'm Vicky and the problem drinker in my life is my daughter."

JOSH

"Hello, my name's Josh and I'm pleased to be here tonight."

JEFF

"My name is Jeff and the person with the drink problem in our life is our son. My wife Alice is here with me tonight. Our son is still drinking and is drunk most days."

INGRID

"Hello, I'm Ingrid and I'm fairly new to the group."

PIPPA

"Hello, I'm Pippa and I'm here tonight because I really need the support I can get from the group."

KALEB

"Hi, I'm Kaleb and the alcoholic in my life is my wife, who is currently trying to give up alcohol without the help of any support group."

ELSA

"Hello I'm Elsa and I am a long time member of the group and it is my father who is the alcoholic in my life".

ALICE

"Hello, my name is Alice and it is our son who has a problem with alcohol."

OLGA

"Hello, I'm Olga and it's nice to see some new faces here tonight. I am a very grateful member of AL even though I don't attend very regularly now."

*   *   *

EDDIE

"Can I remind everyone that this is an anonymous group and we use first names only.

Anonymity is one of the key principles we adhere to in the group.

You do not need to tell us who you are, where you live, where you work, what you do—absolutely nothing about your personal details at all if you don't want to.

There are 12 of us here tonight but the numbers vary each week and sometimes there are more of us and sometimes less.

You don't have to come every week but we do suggest you attend as regularly as you can if you want to benefit from what's on offer here. Our only purpose is to share our experience, strength and hope to help ourselves and each other to gain some peace of mind because our lives have been affected by an alcohol dependent person. Anything else about your life is no concern of ours unless you choose to share it with us.

So, as I've said my name is Eddie and although I am chairing the meeting tonight, next time someone else will be chairing because we practice the principle of rotation of leadership in the group.

A special word for our recent members, it may all still seem strange and you will probably go away not understanding much about what you hear tonight but if you feel something that brings you back then that is enough to be going on with. Just keep coming back and it will eventually start to become much clearer about what support you can gain from the group.

Also, although we meet up in a church hall this programme is not religious and has no connection to any church. The only reason we meet here is because of low costs.

So on with the meeting.

Every week we have a different theme and tonight's theme is:

Looking for Help?

Jeff can you start us off with the 12 steps please?"

JEFF

"Step 1: We admitted we were powerless over the problem drinker and that our lives had become unmanageable."

INGRID

"**Step 2**: We came to believe that a power greater than ourselves could restore us to serenity."

PIPPA

"**Step 3**: We made a decision to turn our will and our lives over to the care of our higher power (HP)."

KALEB

"**Step 4**: We made a searching and fearless moral inventory of ourselves."

ELSA

"**Step 5**: We admitted to our HP, to ourselves and to another human being the exact nature of our wrongs."

ALICE

"**Step 6**: We were entirely ready to have our HP remove all these defects of character."

OLGA

"**Step 7**: We humbly asked our HP to remove our shortcomings."

EDDIE

"**Step 8**: We made a list of all persons we had harmed and became willing to make amends to them all."

STAVROS

"**Step 9**: We made direct amends to such people wherever possible, except when to do so would injure them or others."

CLARISSA

"**Step 10**: We continued to take personal inventory and when we were wrong promptly admitted it."

VICKY

"**Step 11**: We sought through reflection and meditation to improve our conscious contact with our HP, seeking only knowledge of our HP's will for us and the power to carry that out."

JOSH

"**Step 12**: Having had an emotional and spiritual awakening as the result of these Steps, we tried to carry this message to others, and to practice these principles in all our affairs."

*   *   *

EDDIE

"Mack had agreed to be our main sharer for tonight but due to a crisis at home he is unable to be here so Olga has agreed to stand in, at very short notice, to share for us.

Also can I just remind you there is no obligation for anyone to share.

You can remain silent and just listen if you prefer but those who do decide to share are allowed to do so without interruption from others.

So over to you Olga, on the theme of—**Looking for Help?"**

Olga is Russian and it is her ex-husband who was the alcoholic in her life.

OLGA

"Hello, and for the newcomers my name is Olga and I haven't been for a while but I am a very grateful member of AL. There are a few new faces I haven't seen before but I'm sure you will all soon become very familiar to me. The alcoholic in my life was my husband but three years ago he left and 'set up shop' with an ex-friend of mine who was prepared to join him as his drinking buddy. So I sort of lost my husband and my so called best-friend when they decided to move in together and kick me to the curb so to speak. However, I've learned life with an alcoholic can be very, very unpredictable and just a nightmare really so I needed to 'tool myself up' to deal with the challenge I was facing and this group has given me that otherwise I don't know where I would be or what kind of state I would be in now.

Anyway back to tonight's topic, did I look for help? Well, yes I suppose I did after a fashion but it was not very effective for me. The way I went about doing it was all wrong and it just rebounded on me so I think I sort of gave up looking for help and just tried to sort it out myself but my two daughters ended up getting the brunt of my COW behaviour.

Everyone laughs.

Yes, I was a cow, in some ways but that's not what I mean here. I use the acronym COW to illustrate my **C**ontrolling, **O**bsessive, **W**orrying behaviour. If I wasn't trying to control the alcoholic I would switch to worrying over him. If I wasn't worrying about him I would switch to obsessing about his behaviours and so it went on year in, year out but nothing ever changed. I realise now my COW behaviours were just giving me the illusion I was doing something but really I wasn't. My life was circular, controlling, obsessing and worrying but going nowhere.

However, as I was saying in the beginning, I did sort of look for help but I went to the wrong people. I wasn't selective enough. I would talk to colleagues at work, well off-load to them really, rather than have a discussion and I got the kind of advice back that really didn't help me, in fact, I would say it made matters worse. For instance, my boss would say to me 'you want to bloody kick him out' or 'you want to kick him down the bloody stairs' or 'I would have had him out years ago'. I would just listen to all of this but it didn't help me it just added to the burden, trying not to react to this because none of them had a bloody clue what it was really like to live with an active alcoholic.

The duff advice I got just confused me even more than I already was so I think what happened was I just spiralled down into this sort of obsessive thinking pattern so I could never make a decision because I would confide in 3 or 4 different people and they would all say different things so my head became full of duff advice and I would sink into paralysis because of obsessive analysis because I wouldn't know which advice to choose. Then I would try something they had said and it wouldn't work so I would try something else and that wouldn't work either so my self-confidence just ebbed away and I withdrew into myself and I suppose I decided I was alone with the problem and I just had to get on with it the best way I could.

I ended up hiding away from people and lying about how things really were. Holiday times were the worst because when I went back to work the talk would all be about what a fabulous time everyone had had especially at Christmas time but Christmas for me was always an absolute disaster. I couldn't tell people at work that, so I hid it and put a face on and lied about having a nice time just to keep people off my back. The only people in the world who knew what was really going on were my two daughters who were not coping with it very well either but I was too wrapped up in my own controlling, obsessive, worrying behaviours to notice the effect it was having on them.

The image that comes to mind is the impressionist painter Seurat who painted with dots and if you stand up close you only see the dots but if you step back you see the whole landscape and it reminds me of how my relationship with my ex-husband was. I was so embroiled in it that I kept looking closer and closer at him until I was finally looking through a microscope so I couldn't see me in the picture at all because I was too close up. It was only by coming along to AL I heard others share about how they had stepped back and got a clearer view of their situations. I realised I needed to do the opposite of what I had been doing. My instinct had told me to dive in whereas what I could have been doing was getting out of the pool because that's what gave me some clarity to see how things were really working between us. I needed to get a different perspective before I could stop going round in circles.

Out of desperation I turned to my daughters and off-loaded to them, asking for their advice about what to do and this has really backfired on me recently. Now my daughters say I was almost as bad, if not worse, than the alcoholic because at least with him they knew he would just get drunk and fall asleep or whatever but with me I would just go on and on about the problem and it wasn't helped by this obsessive thinking I got into.

In AL we have the slogan '*Think*' but I couldn't think in that situation, everything just became an emotional reaction. I can think today and I can see it was unfair and inappropriate of me to off-load my problems on to people who didn't have the faintest idea how to help. It also made a double problem for me because what would happen is when I asked my daughters for help or other inappropriate people I wouldn't actually be helped I would just end up with two problems instead of one—I would have my original problem then I'd have the problem of my daughters reaction to me asking them for advice. I know now I should not have gone to my children for help but I didn't know any better at the time.

I just used to rant on and on about the problem to my kids because I had isolated myself from the rest of the world and I'd left myself with nobody else to turn to. My kids didn't have the faintest idea what to do, just as I didn't but by that time my thinking had become so narrowed down I couldn't see any other options. I needed to be shown how I could expand my world again.

So I've learned that a 'problem shared can be a problem halved' only if I ask people who can really help but if I ask inappropriate people, which I had a habit of doing, then a problem shared can turn into a problem quadrupled. So now I am much more selective about who I reach out to for help. I don't burden people who really haven't the faintest idea about alcoholism.

Coming to AL was the first time I found any real peace because these people could actually help because they knew the drill and had walked this path before me. So it is AL people who I mostly look to for help because they know and can empathise. So yes, I still do hide the problem but only from people who can't help but with those who can help I do reach out to them.

I am still dealing with the effects all of this crazy behaviour had on my children, having a mother who tried to give them the responsibility of coping with their alcoholic father. I think it will take a long time to sort it out. I was always manic or miserable. I'm pleased to say my knowledge and understanding of alcoholism now gives me the ability to make my own life much more manageable. Thankfully being on the 'Merry-go-Round' is a thing of the past for me, well mostly!

And I will just leave it at that thank you."

GROUP TOGETHER

"Thanks Olga."

JOSH

"Can I come in Eddie?

Josh is in his early twenties and it was his twin-sister who was the alcoholic in his life. She died last year.

Yes, I was looking for help because I was feeling really bad but I had no idea what kind of help or where to find it. Eventually, I ended up going to see a counsellor and she suggested I come here and thank goodness she did because I didn't know anything like this existed for the families of alcoholics. So although it was a bit of a winding road to get here I did eventually find out that the process of recovery was already here in AL but I just had to find it and have the courage to turn up to the meeting—and keep turning up. Thank you."

GROUP TOGETHER

"Thanks Josh."

VICKY

"I'll come in if I may Eddie?

Vicky spent a couple of years sitting in AA meetings in an attempt to manage her alcoholic daughter's drinking problem. When all her efforts failed a few months ago she finally found her way to an AL meeting.

Thanks Olga and Josh for your shares.

Well, I certainly didn't go looking for help. I suppose I was no different from anybody else in this room and a lot of other people in the world because I thought I was the only person who had this problem.

Looking back I didn't know my daughter was an alcoholic I thought she was just going through a phase of heavy drinking and for some reason I just automatically thought I had to hide it, hide it away!

It was almost something I felt I ought to be ashamed of, not necessarily ashamed of my daughter but ashamed of my part in it. I had this nagging question always at the front of my mind, what had I done to make her like this? To me it seemed obvious that it must have been something I had done. Had I not loved her enough? Had I loved her too much? Had I done too much for her when she was a child, yes, but I was no different from most mothers.

So when I first realised she had a problem with alcohol I didn't want to look to anyone for help. I just wanted to fix it myself. I could cope with my life very well but when I think back my time and efforts could have been put to far better use doing something that produced more positive results.

The only other person who knew was her father but I was the one who took charge and became the driving force who could make it all better. I thought I knew best because I'd been making everyone's life better for years so this wasn't any different or so I thought at the time.

I had always been the kind of person who ran around like a 'cat on a hot tin roof' making things better for everyone and I didn't want other people to know about this problem she had. I certainly wanted to shield her grandparents from it. I didn't want them to face the fact their only grand-daughter had all of this going on so I did everything in my power to stop them from finding out.

I suppose I was dealing with the problem myself for about 5 years and I didn't ask anyone for help. I thought I could shoulder the burden and nobody needed to know. When I look back at it now, all I did was make my own life a living hell but I was only focused on the good I thought I was doing by shielding her and everyone else. Eventually, of course it blew up in my face and when it all came out I felt pretty disgusted with myself for all the lies I had told for such a long time because I thought I was helping by doing that.

Apart from the shame, another reason I didn't look for help sooner was because I thought I was a very capable person and I was, but my capabilities were not solving her problem in this situation. It wasn't until she was rushed to hospital and put on a life-support machine because her liver was failing and then obviously the rest of the family found out so I couldn't hide it anymore and it was at that point that everything really came crashing down for me.

Even after she got out of hospital and was admitted to a rehab centre I was still trying to manage her life until I was told to just STOP.

A very experienced nurse at the centre told me to just stop doing what I was doing. It gave me a jolt because that was the first time anyone else had actually started to take the responsibility off my shoulders. She was the first person who told me to think about what I was really doing. I was not really helping I was just making it more comfortable for my daughter to drink and so she would never have any motivation to pick up the responsibility herself.

Yes, she had been in AA but it hadn't been her idea to go. I had frog-marched her there and sat at the back to make sure she stayed. She was doing it for me—not for herself. The nurse told me I couldn't do anything about my daughter's alcohol problem but I could leave her to her AA friends who would know how to help and support her because they could give her the identification she needed which she could never get from me. It seems only alcoholics can really understand other alcoholics. I was just completely devastated but it must have been the right time for me to throw in the towel and accept the reality of my powerlessness over her problem.

I suppose the rest is history, I came along to AL the same week, even though to be perfectly honest, I didn't want to come. I thought everyone here would come from a long way further down the social scale than my family. I thought they would be people who had their backsides hanging out of their trousers and bottles wrapped in brown paper bags sitting on park benches—the lowest of the low really.

Since I came in here I have had a total change of attitude because I have learned there is no such thing as the lowest of the low. We all deserve respect whoever we are and meeting the people here has opened my eyes to that. All alcoholics don't come from rough, deprived places. I was shocked to find out just how much this problem crosses all class barriers, it can affect anybody regardless of how much money they have in the bank or what expensive schools they went to.

So by sitting and listening to everyone I've come to realise there is life out there 'whether the alcoholic is still drinking or not' and in the middle of whatever is going on—I can find peace. Coming to AL is probably the first time I stopped trying to hide the problem and found the courage to not only find, but accept help. When I look back, hiding all of this trouble and struggling on alone, was a very sad thing to do. It was something I did for a long time. I am so pleased I am not in that dark place anymore and I hope I never will be again. They say alcoholism is a black hole for the alcoholic but it can also be a black hole for all of those who love an alcoholic but there is a way to climb out and I think it is by listening to people who have been through it and for that I really thank you all."

GROUP TOGETHER

"Thanks Vicky."

CLARISSA

"Can I come in Eddie?

Clarissa is a woman in her mid-30's who is married to an alcoholic. He had 2 years of sobriety but has occasionally picked up again over the past 6 months.

Thanks everybody for your shares and Olga its lovely to see you back again. As most of you know it's my husband who is the alcoholic in my life and he was a binge drinker I would say for oh about 10 years, easy, maybe more than 10 years and towards the last 2 years of his binge drinking it escalated rapidly until the gap between his drinking was getting down to a couple of days. If he wasn't thinking about a drink he was manoeuvring his way and manipulating his way into a crisis where he could have a drink. So I came here because I was looking for help but I wanted help for him. I wanted him sorted out. It never occurred to me I needed help for myself even though I feared for my own sanity living with him.

I came here and everyone was lovely and they listened to my story and I didn't like it, I hated being here because what I realised after my first few meetings was instead of me trying to find a way to make the alcoholic better I had to start looking at myself and start to improve my life so I would be stronger.

I found out here that no matter how much I tried to analyse the drinking patterns or his way of thinking or manipulation or anything like that, I had absolutely no control over my husband whatsoever and the only person I was chewing up into knots was myself. And I realised the programme, and when I say the programme I mean the 12 steps and the slogans and applying them to my life and keeping the slogans at the forefront of my mind so when a crisis happens, whether it is to do with the alcoholic or just something through the day, I can always bring a slogan into my mind to help me through that rough time.

I found I had to let my husband get on with his own recovery because I was actually hindering him by interfering. Now I know for some of you in here it is a totally different relationship, it can be your child and if one of my children ever started to drink I would be devastated. If that did happen I would have to go right back to the beginning and apply the program to that particular situation but at the moment I just have to apply it to being the wife of an alcoholic and what AL has taught me is that I had to learn to be my own best friend. I had to keep out of the alcoholic's recovery and let him recover at his own pace and I did that by being very disciplined by applying the program everyday to my own life. So I started to do that and gradually I started to get a little bit stronger in myself and it was only after I started to get stronger that I felt like the fog lifted and the anxiety subsided a little bit. I used to sit and shake and didn't sleep and I had a lot of paranoia when I first came here. As I got a little bit stronger all of those started to subside and when the fog lifted a bit I got a clearer view of my situation.

I built up some inner strength through listening to what everybody said, by picking the phone up and speaking to people outside of the meeting. I found the strength to cope with my situation in a calmer, cooler more what's the word I'm looking for?—rational way. But it's not easy and I found I had to keep coming back and practicing *One*

Day at a Time, that for me is my mantra along with *Let Go* and *How important is it?*

For me my HP is the feeling of group, warmth and support I get from the group because once you come to AL you are never alone again with the problem. So that's the way I found help here living *One Day at a Time* and that doesn't mean shrugging off all my responsibilities for the future and for my family it just means I make my plans for the future or the coming week and then I bring my thoughts back and I live in the day and what I found it did for me was it stopped my 'stinking thinking' which was the catastrophising, the what if's?, were in my head all the time and actually when one of the really bad things happened to me, when my husband in a drunken stupor tried to commit suicide. What did I do? I did what was in my power to do, I looked after my three young children. There was nothing I could do about his erratic behaviour and I was told when I came into AL the 3 C's, *No, I didn't cause it, No, I can't control it and No I can't cure it*—because my alcoholic blamed me and eventually I got to the point where I believed him and so my self-esteem was very low and then I was told in here '*No you didn't cause it, No you can't control it and No you can't cure it*' so pack in wasting your time.

It was also suggested I stop analysing everything the alcoholic did and thought, what his next plan was and what he was going to do. Don't try to outwit him by thinking if he does that then I would do this and all that rubbish was driving me towards a nervous breakdown. So *One Day at a Time* I have got better and better and I'm now my own best friend, I have grown and am a stronger person.

I use this programme for every single part of my life now. That's what Step 12 tells me to do—apply these principles in all my affairs, not just the alcoholic situation. So I apply it to my work, my friendships, my relationships, my old 'stinking thinking' when my head goes off it.

Now whenever there is a problem or I'm feeling low or I'm churned up about something in my everyday life, I know I can pick up my programme and apply it to anything. I can apply a slogan, I can pick up the phone and speak to anyone in this room if I want to and it's a wonderful, wonderful way of life and they say it is a programme for life not just for alcoholism and I am glad I'm here and I hope I will be here for a long time to come.

I would say to the newcomers it's not an easy ride so be easy on yourself at the beginning. On my fourth meeting I just kept driving around the block because I didn't want to come in. I didn't want to look at myself, I didn't want to look at the situation, I hated the place and I hated everybody in it suggesting what I should do. Then I thought well Clarissa, you have nowhere else to go if you want to get better, this is about you and retaining some sanity so I parked the car and came back in and I've been coming back ever since. So that's all I've got to say, it's worth sticking around, if you keep an open mind about things because I came here to fix the alcoholic but I stayed to fix me."

GROUP TOGETHER

"Thanks Clarissa."

ELSA

"Can I come in Eddie?

Elsa is the adult child (ACOA) of an alcoholic father. Elsa is a long time member and can speak about her experiences with an air of confidence and emotional detachment which the newer members are unable to do.

For me I think for a long time I didn't ask for help because I was the eldest child and everyone who knew about my Dad kept congratulating me on how well I was coping and I did cope well and I did do a good job. I suppose I thought of myself as some kind of 'Wonderchild' who was living with my alcoholic father and keeping everything together for him. It wasn't until one night I had to ring for yet another ambulance because he'd started to 'fit' and the operator couldn't believe it was a genuine 999 call because I was so calm and 'matter of fact' about my Dad being in such a state she thought I was just a prankster. It took me a long time to convince her that everything was going on just as I said. When the paramedics turned up one of them said to me 'you do know this isn't normal don't you, you do know your reaction is not normal?' and I remember thinking—Is it not? So I wasn't so much keeping my Dad's drinking a secret as I was just doing such a good job everyone had let me get on with it.

This paramedic suggested I talk to someone about me and how my Dad's behaviour had affected my reactions. I found out about AL from one of Dad's drinking friends and it was only when I started talking about it to someone else did I begin to realise, what I thought was normal, absolutely wasn't normal at all, in fact, I had a very abnormal life.

I think until people start to talk more openly about this issue most of it can just go under the radar. I was a child growing up in an alcoholic home and with the best will in the world I just thought I was helping my Dad. It wasn't until I came to this group that I learned I wasn't helping him or any of us really.

It didn't occur to me to question anything I was doing, that was just what I did and it had become very abnormal really. When I was able to talk about it openly I could see I did need help, I couldn't do it all on my own.

I heard in AL that as the eldest child of an alcoholic I had probably developed some really self-sabotaging behaviour patterns in my childhood home. It really helps when things are going through my head and I can't work them out to come in here and share them with others and get suggestions back as to how to cope. I don't expect people to give me an answer but once I get the problem aired it doesn't seem as bad outside my head as it does inside my head. I think part of it is just knowing someone else knows about it helps me a lot.

I know it's only me who can help me but once it is outside of my head either by telling someone or even writing it down it is far easier to manage and cope with. At the time the problem might seem like it's never ending but I can remind myself I have been through worse in the past and have come through it, so I can certainly get through this.

I know sharing it with somebody doesn't mean they have all the answers or a magic pill but my 'what-if's?' were always a hundred times worse than what really happened and people reminded me of that. Even the horrendous things that happened which I didn't imagine I still managed to get through so it was a waste of energy obsessing and worrying so now I can remind myself that This too will Pass and it won't be forever.

I think when people have alcoholism come into their lives they can feel very ashamed to ask for help and they end up trying to hide it but I think as a society we would be much better off being more open and not feel we have to suffer in silence or keep a stiff upper lip about it. It takes a lot of courage to ask for help and I think we should lead by example and not be ashamed of it.

That's all I want to say for now. Thanks Everyone."

GROUP TOGETHER

"Thanks Elsa."

PIPPA

"I'll just quickly share Eddie.

Pippa's boyfriend is the drinker in her life. She came along to the group some time ago but left after a few meetings. She is back because of a current crisis she needs support with.

Well I have had a heck of a week. I'm Pippa and it's my boyfriend who is my lovely alcoholic in my life and I say that because he is a lovely, lovely person when he is not drinking. It's been a rough week with him because I think he's hit a bit of a rock bottom and that's why his drinking is really bad at the minute. He's not in a good place today, in fact, things are so bad, he is in a terrible way. I think it's because of some big changes he's got going on in his life which he feels he has no control over.

I left him because I was finding it very hard going with him drinking all day. The house was full of mayhem as most of you will know, I'm sure I don't have to explain the reasons why I just couldn't handle it."

Pippa is overcome with emotion and stops. She is unable to continue speaking for a while. Everyone sits quietly and waits until she continues with her share.

"I will be totally honest with you all, when I first came to AL a couple of years ago, something like that, I didn't think he was an alcoholic and I still thought I could make him better. I just thought he was a heavy drinker but not an alcoholic. Anyway, when I sat in the meetings I kept looking at people and I came to a few meetings and I thought why are they all so bloody happy? Why are they all laughing their heads off and I've still got all of this crap at home to deal with. I thought good grief, look at them all, one was saying "my one's recovered, another was saying "mine's stopped drinking", someone else was saying "mine hasn't drank for 5 years and when it got to the one who said "mine hasn't drank for 25 years! I though oh it's alright for them, theirs have all stopped drinking mine's still bloody drinking and all the pain I've got and all the anger and annoyance inside of me and I felt quite angry with everybody in the room. I can remember thinking how angry I felt.

Everybody seemed too happy and I felt it wasn't helping me but I realise today these people were in a 'good place' because they had benefitted from coming along regularly to meetings and listened to others who had given them strength. For instance, Clarissa's share last week was out of this world for me, a Gem, and I have taken a lot of strength from that this week. So although I can't stop my boyfriend from drinking I feel as if I am helping him by coming to meetings and trying to stay strong myself. Thanks."

GROUP TOGETHER

"Thanks Pippa."

EDDIE

"I'm mindful of the time but we do have about 5 minutes left if anyone who hasn't already spoken would like to come in and share?"

Eddie makes eye contact with Ingrid and is unsure as to whether or not she would like to share.

"Would you like to come in Ingrid?"

Ingrid is a relatively new member to the AL Group. It's her husband who is alcohol dependent.

INGRID

"No Eddie, I would just like to sit quietly and listen tonight, thanks."

GROUP TOGETHER

"Thanks Ingrid."

STAVROS

"I will just quickly come in Eddie?"

The alcoholic in Stavros' life was his wife. He does not know whether she is still alive or not. The last time he heard any news of her, she was spotted living on the streets but he has never been able to track her down.

"Just going back to something Pippa said about all the smiling faces she saw when she first came along to the meeting. I can certainly identify with that because I also felt very annoyed with all the Cheshire Cat smiles I got when I first walked in. I thought these people cannot be for real!

I thought maybe this was some loony new-age stuff and I kept my distance for quite a few months and quickly disappeared as soon as the meeting finished to avoid having any conversations with anybody. Eventually, I came to realise all these people were dealing with the same thing I was and somehow they were happy and I got to thinking how the heck are they doing that? It was a new thing for me seeing happy people. I heard people saying they felt the comfort and hope in the room and I thought OK what can I do to get that?

I started by making little changes and doing things they were doing to be more serene. It took a long time for me to loosen up and relax enough to listen carefully to what others were saying because I felt like smacking some of them in the mouth, that's how affected I had become by living with alcoholism for so many years.

One thing I did like was the slogan *'Take what you like and leave the rest'* because it made me feel more comfortable knowing I could test out what worked for me and leave anything which I didn't like and that's what I've done and it works for me. Today I can look back at those early days and laugh at myself and it gives me a great sense of happiness just seeing how far I've come since those wilderness years. Thanks."

GROUP TOGETHER

"Thanks Stavros."

EDDIE

"So it's that time again so can I just remind our recent members we suggest you come back for at least 6 meetings before you decide whether it's for you or not. The reason we say that is because we have different members and different topics here at different times and it could be that you don't find anyone you feel you can identify with at your first few meetings.

However, if after 6 meetings you find no identification then the group is probably either not for you or not for you at this time.

Before we close our meeting tonight I will just remind everybody of the theme for next time is—

Reacting

Do we have a volunteer to be the main sharer for next time?"

STAVROS

"I will be the main sharer Eddie."

EDDIE

"Thank You Stavros.

So it just remains for me to say that there are no dues for membership but we do ask you to make a contribution of whatever you can afford to cover our costs for tea and coffee and rent. If you cannot afford anything then that is OK too.

OK, I'm afraid our time is up and we close on time, so Alice, can I ask you to read the suggested closing to close our meeting please?"

ALICE

"In closing, I would like to say that the opinions expressed here were strictly those of the person who gave them. Take what you liked and leave the rest. A few words to those of you who haven't been with us long: whatever your problems, there are those amongst us who have had them too. If you try to keep an open mind, you will find help.

You will come to realise that there is no situation too difficult to be bettered and no unhappiness too great to be lessened.

Will all those who care to join me in closing our meeting?"

Everyone joins hands in a circle.

GROUP TOGETHER

"Grant me the Serenity to accept the things I cannot change.
The courage to change the things I can and
The wisdom to know the difference.
Same time, Same Place, Keep coming back, it works if you work it."

www.ingramcontent.com/pod-product-compliance
Lightning Source LLC
Chambersburg PA
CBHW021241280526
45784CB00005B/2184